How-to Guide for Cialis

Beyond The Pill: Lasting-Long Erection Pills for Men, Acting Fast, Get and Stay Rock Hard, Pure Mind-Blowing Climax

Dr. Alma Rodrigues

Copyright @

All rights reserved. Except for brief quotes used in critical reviews and other noncommercial purposes allowed by copyright law, no part of this publication may be reproduced, distributed, or transmitted in any form by any means, electronic, mechanical, photocopying, recording, or otherwise.

DISCLAIMER

This content of this book should only be used for general educational and informative purposes. It should not be used in place of an expert medical advice, diagnosis or care. In fact, you should always consult your healthcare provider if you have any questions about a medical issue

Table of Contents

Copyright @ 1

Chapter One 4
    Introduction 4

Chapter Two 10
    Taking Cialis 10

Chapter Three 13
    Using Cialis 13

Chapter Four 20
    Side Effects 20

Chapter Five 26
    Those who can't take Cialis 26

Chapter Six 28
    Precautions 28

Chapter Seven 32
    Interactions 32

Chapter Eight 36
    Overdose 36
        Cialis Overdose Symptoms 37
        Overdose Treatment 38
        Overdose Prevention 39
        Taking Care of a Missed Dose 42

Chapter Nine 43
    Storage of Cialis 43

The End 44

Chapter One

Introduction

This book can help if you're looking for a cure for erectile dysfunction issues.

The inability to achieve or sustain an erection has been deemed important by medical specialists, and Cialis (tadalafil) is one of the medications that is most frequently recommended to treat it.

Tadalafil is used to treat erectile dysfunction, a condition that affects male sexual performance. This drug belongs to the group of pharmaceuticals called phosphodiesterase 5 (PDE5) inhibitors.

These drugs cause phosphodiesterase type-5 to stop working too soon. The penis is one area where this enzyme is active.

Erectile dysfunction is the term used to describe a man's inability to sustain an erection after experiencing six sexual thrills. Tadalafil prolongs an erection by controlling the enzyme, while a man's body naturally increases blood flow to his penis in response to sexual stimulation. In the absence of physical stimulus to the penis, such as that which occurs during sexual intercourse, tadalafil will not cause an erection.

Tadalafil can also be used to treat men who show signs and symptoms of benign prostatic hyperplasia (BPH). An enlarged condition is the root cause of BPH. Benign prosthetic hyperplasia (BPH) in males usually causes lower pee flow at the beginning of the flow, difficulty voiding, and midnight urination.

Tadalafil may diminish the intensity of symptoms and reduce the need for potential prostate surgery. This drug is also used to treat erectile dysfunction and BPH symptoms.

Tadalafil is also prescribed to men and women to treat the symptoms of pulmonary arterial hypertension and to increase their capacity for activity.

The main blood vessel from the ventricle on the right side of the heart is impacted by this hypertension. When the smaller blood vessels in the lungs become more resistant to blood flow, the right ventricle must work harder to pump blood through the lungs. Tadalafil works on the PDE5 enzyme in the lungs to relax blood vessels.

The heart will therefore pump more blood to the lungs while exerting less effort.

Tadalafil was approved by the US Food and Drug Administration (USFDA) in 2003 as a treatment for erectile dysfunction.

Cialis and other PDE5 inhibitors do not improve low libido or erectile dysfunction. However, drugs must be used both physically and psychologically in order to aid in achieving and maintaining an erection.

When the parasympathetic nervous system is activated, as happens during sexual desire, nitric oxide (NO) is released. Greater cyclic GMP production is a result of high NO levels. Because Cialis for ED relaxes the arteries feeding the penis, more blood can enter it. Because Essien relaxes the muscles in the bladder, it becomes simpler to urinate and lessens the signs and symptoms of BPH. Cialis may only be purchased with a prescription.

Chapter Two
Taking Cialis

During a penile erection, blood swells the penis. This is because unrestricted blood flow is made possible by the veins feeding the penis. The blood vessels coming from the penis deteriorate as a result. An erection happens when the penis fills with blood.

As part of its mechanism of action, Cialis also blocks the effects of a prescription drug that the body commonly carries into the penis during sexual activity. Consequently, the stream design can now get close to the penis. An increase in blood flow to specific inside penile areas is typically the source of erections.

Nitric oxide eventually reaches the penis, where it gives a guy a sense of desirability.

The blood vessels that supply and drain the penis are controlled by cGMP and nitric oxide. An alternative atom that performs better than cGMP is PDE5. Now that the erection is over, the veins go back to their resting position. PDE5 is not able to outperform cGMP when taking Cialis. An erection that lasts longer could come from this.

This pharmacological method may help treat pneumonic hypertension because PDE5 is found in the muscles surrounding the lungs' dividing veins.

Chapter Three

Using Cialis

Cialis comes as yellow, film-coated, almond-shaped pills ranging from 5 to 20 mg. A prescription medication called Cialis is used to treat male sexual dysfunction, or erectile dysfunction (ED). Tadalafil increases blood flow to the penis, which aids in a man's ability to get and maintain an erection when accompanied with sexual stimulation. When taken without any kind of sexual stimulation, this medication does not produce erections. The right circumstances have to be fulfilled for the medication to take effect when it is activated.

Weak streams, frequent urges to urinate, and trouble starting the flow of urine during urination are all signs of BPH. Another drug used to treat such symptoms is tadalafil. It is well known that tadalafil causes the smooth muscles of the prostate and bladder to relax.

Moreover, it has no effect on HIV, syphilis, gonorrhea, or hepatitis B, which are communicable diseases. Consult your physician or pharmacist for additional information. Read the Patient Information Leaflet that your doctor gave you before beginning to use tadalafil. Next, read it once more before each refill. See your primary care physician or another medical expert if you have any concerns. Take this drug orally, as prescribed by your physician, either with or without food. It is recommended to use tadalafil just once day. Whether you take drugs, how well you respond to treatment, and the severity of your condition will all affect the estimate. To find out more information about the medications you are taking, speak with a pharmacist or your primary care physician. This covers over-the-counter pharmaceuticals, prescription drugs, and everyday items.

There are two dosages for Cialis. You can get advice from your doctor on the best way to take Cialis. Because the way you take your prescription affects the dose, be sure you follow your doctor's recommendations carefully. For the first technique, a starting dose of 10 mg should be given half an hour before sexual activity. After taking tadalafil, sexual activity may be affected for up to 36 hours. The patient's response may then dictate a change in the dosage. In any event, a single 20 mg dose is the most drastic method. It is allowed to take one dose per 24 hours. However, because drug fragments can remain in the bloodstream for up to 24 hours, a daily dose of 10–20 mg is not advised.

Patients may take 5 mg twice weekly if they want to participate in active, dynamic behavior (like sexual activity); however, the amount may be reduced to 2.5 mg based on the patient's response.

For erectile dysfunction, Cialis is a prescription medication available to both men and women over the age of 18.

Regular Cialis use is the next stage in curing erectile dysfunction. You can have sex whenever you want if you have it often. Use this medication as prescribed by your doctor once daily to treat the symptoms of BPH. If you're taking finasteride to treat the symptoms of BPH, consult your pharmacist or doctor about the right dosage and duration of use.

As prescribed, take one dose of Cialis per day if you have erectile dysfunction along with BPH. Intermittent periods are acceptable for sexual engagement.

To treat ED, BPH, or both, take the drug every day. It's advised that you use recurring reminders to assist in remembering to take your medication. If things don't get better or get worse, schedule a visit with your doctor.

Chapter Four
Side Effects

Taking a nitrate supplement along with tadalafil or Cialis will significantly lower your blood pressure, a condition known as hypotension.

Cialis should not be taken if you are using a nitrate for chest discomfort or heart issues.

If any of the following indications of true complexity appear during intercourse, get medical help right away:

- Migraine
- Constipation
- Backache

- Aches and pains in the muscles
- Nose blockage
- Flushing
- Dizziness

Please get in touch with your primary care physician or a pharmaceutical expert right once if any of these side effects worsen or persist.

You can reduce your chances of feeling exhausted and confused by getting up gradually from a sitting or sleeping position.

Recall that your doctor prescribed this medication because there are more benefits than drawbacks. Very few side effects are experienced by a large number of users of this medication.

Engaging in sexual activity can significantly worsen heart strain if you already have heart issues. You should immediately stop having sex and see a doctor if you experience any of the following symptoms in addition to heart issues.

- Dazedness.
- Swooning,
- Chest Ache
- Jaw ache
- Pains in the arms.
- Nausea

Rarely, an abrupt loss of vision in one or both eyes can lead to long-term visual impairment (NAION). If this risky circumstance arises, stop taking tadalafil and get medical help right away. Your risk of NAION is somewhat increased if you smoke, have high blood pressure, diabetes, high cholesterol, certain other eye conditions ("crowded disk"), hypertension, or are older than 50.

On rare occasions, a person may have an abrupt loss of hearing, possibly accompanied by ear ringing and vertigo. Should you have any of these adverse effects, stop taking Tadalafil right once and see a physician.

You should cease taking this medication as soon as possible and get medical help if you experience an uncomfortable or delayed erection that lasts more than four hours. You run the danger of running into issues again if you don't.

Serious hypersensitivity responses are rare when using this medication. If you get a rash, tingling or swelling (particularly on the face, tongue, or throat), extreme wooziness, or trouble falling asleep, get emergency medical attention.

The results are by no means all-inclusive. If you have any other unpleasant side effects not on this list, speak with a medication expert or your primary care physician.

Chapter Five
Those who can't take Cialis

Only with your doctor's approval and prescription can you use Cialis if you have any of the following conditions:

- infection of the liver or kidneys.
- an ulcer in the digestive system.
- anything that prevents individuals from having sexual connections.
- One can take many readings of their blood pressure. Leukemia, myeloma, leukopenia, sickle cell anemia,

hemophilia, and other blood disorders can affect individuals.
- One kind of retinitis that affects the eyes is called retinitis pigmentosa.
- Within the recent three or six months, you experienced a stroke, congestive heart failure, or myocardial dead tissue. For instance, Peyronie's illness alters the structure of the penis. Think about angina or any type of cardiac condition.

Chapter Six

Precautions

Before taking Cialis, let your doctor or pharmacist know if you have ever experienced hypertension or any other sensitivity. This product may include inactive chemicals that lead to hypertension and other health issues. Speak with your pharmacist or a professional for more details.

Talk to your doctor or pharmacist about your medical history, particularly if you have experienced any of the following conditions: high or low blood pressure, liver disease, kidney disease, penis conditions (such as fibrosis/scarring, angulation, Peyronie's disease), cardiovascular breakdown, chest pain/angina, stroke in the last six months, or a history of problematic or delayed erections (priapism).

Dizziness is an adverse effect of tadalafil. Both alcohol and marijuana have the potential to make you drunk. Wait until you are sure you can complete the task safely before using any equipment, operating a vehicle, or doing any other action that demands availability. Use of it shouldn't be widespread.

Consult your physician before consuming marijuana.

Talk to your doctor or a dental professional about all medications you take before surgery (including over-the-counter goods, prescriptions written by professionals, and medications recommended by non-specialists).

Women are not supposed to use this drug. Use it only when absolutely necessary when pregnant. Before taking any medication, talk with your doctor about its advantages and disadvantages.

Ascertain with your physician before nursing as to whether this drug is excreted in breast milk.

Chapter Seven

Interactions

Drug interactions have the potential to seriously harm you or change how well your medications work. By no means is this a comprehensive list. Make a list of everything you use, including over-the-counter, prescription, and herbal supplements. You should talk about this list with both your primary care physician and a pharmaceutical expert. Starting, stopping, or switching medications without first talking to your primary care physician is never a wise choice. Riociguat is one medication that might interact with this one.

Tadalafil can dramatically drop blood pressure when combined with nitrates, which raises the risk of fainting, blackouts, and, in rare instances, coronary failure or stroke. Use tadalafil with caution if you are taking nitrates (nitroglycerine, isosorbide), sports drugs that contain butyl or amyl nitrite, or some angina therapies.

Your pulse may drop too low if you use an alpha blocker (doxazosin or tamsulosin, for example, to treat BPH or hypertension) and have dizziness or blackout. Your primary care physician may change the alpha blocker you take or lower the amount of tadalafil you take to lower the risk of low blood pressure.

Depending on the prescription, tadalafil may exit your body in a different method, which could impact how well it works. Examples include rifampin, boceprevir and telaprevir for hepatitis C, itraconazole, ketoconazole, macrolide antibiotics erythromycin and clarithromycin, and HIV protease inhibitors ritonavir and fosamprenavir.

Avoid taking tadalafil or similar medications (vardenafil, sildenafil, etc.) while using this medication if you have pulmonary hypertension or erectile dysfunction.

Chapter Eight
Overdose

The primary component of Cialis, tadalafil, helps to sustain strong erections. Overdoses on Cialis have been documented, however they can occasionally occur by accident. When this medicine is used excessively, side effects and symptoms may occur. Go to the closest emergency center or get in touch with your social insurance provider right away if you think you may have overdosed on a prescription medication.

Cialis Overdose Symptoms

The following warning indicators of a Cialis overdose should be recognized by you:

- Chest pain from anxiety
- Heartbeat Disruption
- Dizziness
- Having trouble remaining awake or experiencing dizziness
- Nausea

Moreover, it might make negative reactions like this more likely.

- Headaches
- Indigestion
- Sterilization of cosmetics
- Back pain

- A strained muscle
- The obstruction of the nasal passages is known as nasal congestion.
- Arms and legs are especially achy.

There may be more symptoms that are not included in this manual.

Overdose Treatment

As soon as possible, sedative overdoses must be reported so that the right care can be given. The restorative administrations provider will suggest a course of treatment based on the indications and symptoms of prescription usage. A Cialis overdose is not treated with a particular medication. The majority of the time, treatment involves ongoing mental tasks.

Overdose Prevention

Keep in mind that Cialis can linger in your system for up to 72 hours to prevent an overdose. Patients should typically take one Cialis pill each day. Continuous dosage and dosing as needed are the two distinct dose techniques. Consult your physician or pharmacist for precise dosage instructions, and thoroughly read the medication label. Ask your pharmacist any questions you may have about the medication or the suggested course of treatment.

Follow the medication's instructions to the letter. Avoid self-medicating if the medication isn't helping or if you need it to start working right away. Think on how Cialis barely affects erections. It could aid in achieving an erection if you're experiencing extreme euphoria.

Avoiding anything that can obstruct Cialis's processing or mode of action is also a smart idea. For example, patients should not consume grapefruits or grapefruit juice. The body could not be able to metabolize

Cialis due to the grapefruit content, which could lead to an overdose. Use Cialis three days or more after taking grapefruit juice.

Cialis shouldn't be taken with other medications for erectile dysfunction, such as vardenafil (Levitra) or sildenafil (Viagra). Make sure you've thought of every scenario before responding. Since only one in eight people are affected by these diseases, each patient needs specialized care.

Taking Care of a Missed Dose

Should you frequently forget to take your medication, take it as soon as you remember. Don't take the missed dose if the next one is almost due. Eat your next meal at the same time every day to make up for lost time.

Chapter Nine
Storage of Cialis

Store it at room temperature, out of direct sunlight, and dry. Never use the bathroom as a place to store things. There should never be drug availability for kids or animals.

Drugs should not be disposed of or dumped into the sink or toilet unless directed otherwise. Please dispose of this item responsibly once it has expired or is no longer needed.

The End